The Complete Salt cure

How consumption Might retain Your essence and promote good vascular health

By

Richard E. Davis

Introduction

Health Benefits: Why We Need Salt in Our Diet — but Not Too Much

It's brilliant to watch out for how much salt is in your eating routine, as suggested by the Dietary Rules for Americans. Individuals over the age of 14 ought to consume something like 2,300 mg each day. Be that as it may, don't keep away from salt completely, as this mineral is a significant part of your body's capabilities. You

want something like 500 mg of sodium (somewhat less than ¼ teaspoon) each day

, On the off chance that the sodium levels in your blood are deficient — a condition called hyponatremia — it very well may be hazardous. Here is a gander at why you want salt in your eating routine:

To Help Your Thyroid Function Properly

Your thyroid assumes a significant part in digestion. Be that as it may, for your thyroid to work appropriately, your body needs the mineral iodine, which is tracked down in numerous food varieties

., iodine lack keeps your body from delivering enough of the thyroid chemical. Side effects of

inadequacy incorporate a developed thyroid, obstruction, trouble thinking, exhaustion, and aversion to cold. Since iodine is added to many salts (marked "iodized"), having some iodized salt in your eating regimen can help your thyroid capability appropriately. Handled food varieties and specialty salts ordinarily don't contain iodine, as the NIH indicates.

To Stay Hydrated

Sodium additionally advances solid hydration levels and electrolyte balance, which is fundamental for your body to work appropriately. Your cells, muscles, and tissues need water, and salt assists these pieces of your body with keeping up with the perfect proportion of liquid,

To Improve Symptoms of Cystic Fibrosis

Individuals living with cystic fibrosis lose more salt in their sweat than the typical individual. According to the Cystic Fibrosis Establishment, they need more water and salt in their eating routine to avoid a lack of hydration. If you have this condition, counsel your primary care physician to perceive how much salt you want daily, founded on your movement level.

Chapter 1

High blood pressure and salt

Salt has been utilized to flavor and safeguard food varieties for millennia. We, as a whole, need some salt for good wellbeing; however, eating in excess can expand our circulatory strain, expanding our gamble of coronary illness. Here we talk about how excessive salt can increment circulatory strain, the connection between salt and Hypertension across Europe, and how we might diminish our salt admission.

What is salt?

Salt is the common name for sodium chloride (or NaCl). It comprises 40% sodium and 60% chloride. 2.5 g of salt contains 1 g of sodium and 1.5 g of chloride.

Why do we need salt?

Both sodium and chloride are fundamental for the overwhelming majority of body capabilities. They assist with directing circulatory strain, controlling liquid equilibrium, keeping up with the right circumstances for muscle and nerve capability, and considering the assimilation and transport of supplements across cell layers. Chloride is additionally used to deliver stomach corrosive (hydrochloric corrosive, HCl), which assists us with processing food varieties.

How much salt do we need per day?

The specific least day-to-day prerequisite for salt is obscure. However, it is believed to be around 1.25 g - 2.5 g (0.5 - 1 g sodium) per day.1 As salt is found in an enormous assortment of food varieties, the gamble of lack is low.1,2 The European Food Handling Authority (EFSA) has expressed that a salt admission of 5 g each day (comparable to 2 g of sodium) is adequate to meet our sodium and chloride necessities and decrease our gamble of Hypertension and heart disease. This is identical to around one teaspoon of salt from all sources daily.

Both sodium and chloride are let out of our body through our pee and when we sweat. This implies episodes of heavy perspiring, for example, during activity, can expand our salt prerequisites marginally. Be that as it may, as many people consume well above the required levels, it is typically not essential to increment salt admission during these conditions.

How much salt do people eat in Europe?

The regular admission of salt fluctuates across Europe, going from 8 to 12 g daily. Consume well above suggested levels. Men will frequently devour more salt than ladies as they will more often than not eat more food, generally speaking.

What is blood pressure?

Circulatory strain is the proportion of the heart's power to siphon blood around the body. There are two measures: systolic circulatory strain (the most noteworthy tension on veins when the heart pushes blood out) and diastolic pulse (the slightest pressure on veins when the heart unwinds between pulsates). Both are estimated in millimeters of mercury (mmHg) and are often introduced as a proportion of systolic/diastolic (for example, 120/80 mmHg).

As a general rule, good circulatory strain is believed to be between 90/60 mmHg and 120/80 mmHg.

Hypertension (otherwise called Hypertension) is often characterized as an estimation of 140/90mmHg or higher. It is a gamble factor for some infections, particularly coronary illness and stroke.

How standard is high blood pressure (Hypertension) in Europe?

In 2015, an expected 1.13 billion individuals were living with Hypertension all around the world, of which 150 million were living in Europe (roughly 23.2% of the population).4 Albeit the pervasiveness (% of the number of inhabitants in) Hypertension in numerous European nations has diminished somewhat as of late, current levels are still of great concern. Diminishing salt admission is a significant general wellbeing methodology to diminish levels further.

Similarly, as with salt admission, the pervasiveness of Hypertension will generally be higher for men than for ladies (figure 2). The specific justification for this distinction isn't wholly perceived; however, higher admissions of salt might be part of the way to a fault.

How does salt increase our blood pressure?

Ordinarily, our kidneys control the sodium and water levels of our blood. Be that as it may, for the overwhelming majority of us, eating an excessive amount of salt can upset this equilibrium, causing sodium levels in the blood to increment. This leads our body to clutch more water and increments both the liquid encompassing our cells and the volume of blood in our circulatory system. As blood volume presses, our veins start to increment, and our heart needs to work harder to move blood around our body. Over the long run, this additional strain can prompt solidifying of veins and expands the gamble of Hypertension, coronary illness, and stroke.

Does reducing salt improve our blood pressure?

There is predictable proof that moderate decreases (for example, a diminishing of 3 to 5 g or ½ to 1 teaspoon daily) in salt admission can prompt a drop in blood pressure.5,6 Be that as it may, these impacts may not be any different for everybody and will rely upon a singular's beginning circulatory strain (more prominent advantages are found in those with worse Hypertension), their ebb and flow level of salt admission, hereditary qualities, sickness status, and prescription use.

It is essential to take note that salt isn't the primary way of life factor that can impact our circulatory strain. Different factors like eating sufficient potassium, keeping a solid body weight, not smoking, and being genuinely dynamic are also significant regarding diminishing circulatory strain.

Chapter 2

The war against salt

Salt of the Sea or the Table?

Here is the thing about salt: there are various types. Keeping in mind that they are very similar, they are likewise divergent in a few critical divisions. It is essential to have the option to distinguish these to appropriately focus on yourself.

The vast majority of us work with table salt daily, and it is acquired through mining salt stores. It is typically strengthened with iodine which is fundamental for thyroid chemical creation. Table salt goes through an interaction that strips it of its minerals to make a delicate surface, invigorates it with this iodine, and is given added substances to forestall clustering. In this manner, it is the best cooking and sprinkling salt; it blends easily.

Ocean salt, then again, is acquired straightforwardly through the dissipation of seawater. It has practically zero handling, and subsequently, it holds follow levels of regular minerals like magnesium, potassium, calcium, iron, and others. Be that as it may, it has no iodine. Assuming you see ocean salt versus table salt as a result of the sodium, remember that it is finished by weight and that ocean salt is more excellent. All salts are 40% sodium by weight.

Salt is made up of two things: sodium and chloride.

Here is the thing about salt: there are various types. Keeping in mind that they are very similar, they are likewise divergent in a few critical divisions. It is essential to have the option to distinguish these to appropriately focus on yourself.

Sodium is a fundamental supplement that drives L-ascorbic acid to the cerebrum, controls circulatory strain, assists nerve and muscle with working, advances ordinary cell capability, permits upkeep of corrosive equilibrium in the blood, and balances destructive mineral irregular characteristics to help thyroid capability. Fundamentally, it does a smidgen of all that, which is why it is fundamental. While the vast majority of this can be tended to with any piece of sodium, not all contain iodine as most table salts do. Continuously ensure you see iodine on the mark while buying, as consuming this kind of salt can assist you with staying away from a lack of iodine which can cause development and mental problems in kids, goiter, and different side effects.

Curb Your Cravings: Sweet or Salty?

Many people are nervous about contacting salt because we correspond it with sugar. We discuss it when we talk about how we taste things, what we hunger for, and the prizes both proposition us when consumed. The issue here is sugar doesn't bring anything to the table for us as salt does.

It could happen for a very long time how destructive sugar is. Yet, tragically, I'm similarly as delicate to these desires as anyone else and should not be reprimanding anybody for this enslavement. They make it hard to move away from it. Be that as it may trust me, go home for the week from eating sugar and see how it treats your body and psyche. I dare you. Particularly on the off chance that you don't genuinely think pulling out from food can impersonate pulling out from a medication. It's revolting.

However, here is the thing about salt. Salt doesn't cause you to hunger for more salt than sugar does. Sweet taste receptors don't flag for you to quit eating desserts. They cause you to hunger for more sugar, and for that reason, it is so hazardous.

Salt taste receptors "flip" when you eat heaps of it and give you an abhorrence signal. This implies your body has an underlying protection instrument that makes you hunger for less salt during the day in the wake of consuming a great deal of it.

Contemplate how you feel after eating a heap of Chinese food or pizza. Furthermore, the delightful thing about salt? Unlike sugar, the less you eat it, the less you want. Along these lines, if you are looking to ween yourself off your sodium diet, you can. What's more, you'll discover that salt is a mixed bag, and when you eat less, you endure less and the other way around.

Food for Thought…

Eat more fresh food.

Foods grown from the ground are generally low in sodium. At the same time, handled food varieties like bread, bagels, pizza, lunch meats, cheddar, soups, cheap food, and arranged suppers with pasta and heart are exceptionally high in sodium. Genuine entire food varieties that are new or frozen poultry or meat have not been infused with sodium-containing arrangements and have the usually happening sodium that you do need. Become a close acquaintance with your butcher! You can trust them to tell you how to find grass-took care of meat, and new wild-gotten fish.

Beware of False Labels!

Continuously view nourishment realities on the back as a great deal of handled and canned food varieties are mislabeled by a showcasing group putting forth a valiant effort to make a powerful check. I will get more into this later; however, think about the way that "low-sodium" commercials on rice boxes imply that they are worse for you than plain-long grain rice.

Condiments Are Silent Killers

Soy sauce, salad dressings, plunges, ketchup, and so forth have a few wild fixings in them and contain a great deal of garbage that we disregard with stacks of sodium we don't consider. Think about it. I have been getting a charge out of Imprint Sisson's Basic Kitchen line as I feel he is somebody considering my wellbeing when I feel the requirement for a dressing I can feel significantly better about that has not many fixings and just purposes entire food varieties and extra-virgin olive oil.

Spice Up Your Life

Try not to underrate the advantages of preparing your food with new and dry spices. Maybe you get a cultivating propensity simultaneously! Continuously consider adding your flavors and spices that have just their name on the rundown of fixings. Use zing and juice from a genuine natural product. It goes pretty far, and you can't beat the kind of real food and plants.

Chapter 3

What causes heart diseases

What is heart disease?

Coronary illness is some of the time called coronary illness (CHD). It's the main source of death among grown-ups in the U.S. Finding out about the causes and hazard variables of the infection might assist you with keeping away from heart issues.

What are the causes of heart disease?

Coronary illness happens when plaque creates in the supply routes and veins that lead to the heart. This blocks effective supplements and oxygen from arriving at your core.

Plaque is a waxy substance comprised of cholesterol, greasy particles, and minerals. Plaque aggregates over the long run when the internal covering of a supply route is harmed by Hypertension, cigarette smoking, or raised cholesterol or fatty substances.

What are the risk factors of heart disease?

A few gambling factors assume a significant part in deciding if you're probably going to foster coronary illness. Two of these variables, age, and heredity, are beyond your control.

The gamble of coronary illness increments around the age of 55 in ladies and 45 in men. Your risk might be more noteworthy on the off chance that you have close relatives who have a background marked by coronary illness.

Other gamble factors for coronary illness include:

• corpulence

• insulin obstruction or diabetes

• elevated cholesterol and circulatory strain

• family background of coronary illness

• being genuinely dormant

• smoking

• eating an unfortunate eating regimen

• clinical discouragement

The link between heart disease and type 2 diabetes

The Public Establishment of Diabetes and Stomach related and Kidney Infections gauges that individuals with type 2 diabetes — and particularly the individuals who have arrived at middle age — are two times as liable to have a coronary illness or experience a stroke as individuals who don't have diabetes.

Grown-ups with diabetes will more often than not have cardiovascular failures at a younger age. They're bound to encounter other cardiovascular defeats on the off chance that they have insulin obstruction or high blood glucose levels.

The justification behind this is the connection between glucose and vein well-being.

High blood glucose levels that aren't overseen can expand how much plaque structures inside the veins' walls. This frustrates or stops the progression of blood to the heart.

If you have diabetes, you can decrease the gamble of coronary illness by dealing with your glucose cautiously. Follow a diabetes-accommodating eating routine that is wealthy in fiber and low in sugar, fat, and straightforward starches. Dealing with your glucose levels can likewise assist with removing your gamble for an eye infection and dissemination issues.

You ought to likewise keep a solid weight. Furthermore, on the off chance you smoke, this present time's a decent opportunity to think about halting.

Discouragement and coronary illness

A few investigations have shown that individuals with discouragement foster coronary illness at higher rates than everybody.

Discouragement can prompt various changes in your body that can expand your gamble of creating coronary illness or cardiovascular failure. Excessive pressure, reliably feeling miserable, or both can hoist your circulatory strain.

Furthermore, discouragement raises levels of a substance called C-responsive protein (CRP). CRP is a marker for irritation in the body. Higher than ordinary degrees of CRP have additionally been displayed to anticipate coronary illness.

Discouragement may likewise prompt a diminished interest in day-to-day exercises. This incorporates daily schedules like an activity that is important to assist with forestalling coronary illness. Other undesirable ways of behaving may follow, for example,

• skipping prescriptions

• not investing energy into eating a sound eating regimen

• drinking an excessive amount of liquor

• smoking cigarettes

Converse with your primary care physician on the off chance that you suspect you have discouragement. Professional assistance can get you back on the way to great well-being and may diminish the possibility of repeating issues.

Coronary illness is hazardous; however, it may be generally forestalled. Everybody would profit from keeping a heart-solid way of life. However, it's especially significant for those with expanded risk.

Prevent heart disease by doing the following:

• Work out consistently.

• Keep a sound eating regimen.

• Keep a good weight.

• Diminish pressure in your life.

• Quit smoking.

• Drink with some restraint.

• Get actual yearly tests from your primary care physician to distinguish irregularities and evaluate risk factors.

• Take supplements, as encouraged by your primary care physician.

• Know the admonition indications of coronary illness, cardiovascular failure, and stroke.

Carrying on with a reliable way of life is quite possibly the best way you can forestall coronary illness, cardiovascular failure, and stroke. Focus on forestalling coronary disease, whether in your 20s or 60s.

Chapter 4

How much salt do we need?

The American Heart Affiliation suggests something like 2,300 milligrams (mg) a day and pushes toward an ideal restriction of something like 1,500 mg each day for most grown-ups.

Since the typical American eats such a lot of overabundance sodium, in any event, scaling back by 1,000 milligrams daily can fundamentally further develop circulatory strain and heart wellbeing.

Furthermore, recollect, more than 70% of the sodium Americans eat comes from bundled, ready, and café food varieties — not the salt shaker.

By and large, Americans eat more than 3,400 milligrams of sodium every day — substantially more than the American Heart Affiliation and other wellbeing associations suggest. The vast majority of us are reasonably underrating how much sodium we eat on the off chance that we can appraise it by any stretch of the imagination.

Holding sodium under tight restraints is essential for following a clever dieting design.

How can I tell how much sodium I'm eating?

You can find sodium in your food by peering at the Nourishment Realities mark. How much is sodium per serving recorded in milligrams (or mg)? Check the fixing list for words like "sodium," "salt," and "pop." The absolute sodium displayed on the Nourishment Realities mark incorporates the sodium from salt and the sodium from some other sodium-containing fixing in the item. For instance, this contains fixings like sodium nitrate, sodium citrate, monosodium glutamate (MSG) or sodium benzoate.

Make sure to observe the serving size on the Nourishment Realities mark. If your piece size rises to two servings of an item, you're eating twofold the sodium recorded.

Here are sodium-related terms you may see on food packages:

• Salt/Without sodium - Under 5 milligrams of sodium for every serving

• Exceptionally Low Sodium - 35 milligrams or less per serving

• Low Sodium - 140 milligrams or less per serving

• Diminished Sodium - Somewhere around 25% less sodium per serving than the standard sodium level

• Light in Sodium or Delicately Salted-Somewhere around 50% less sodium than the customary item

No-Salt-Added or Unsalted - No salt is added during handling - however, these items may not be salt/without sodium except if expressed

Keep in mind: Sodium levels fluctuate in similar food varieties depending upon the brand or eatery.

By the day's end, it's not difficult to count how much sodium you consumed, so you can settle on better decisions depending on the situation. Some of the time, a slight change can bring enormous outcomes with regard to your wellbeing!

Is there such a thing as eating too little sodium?

Stressed that you're not getting sufficient sodium? It's not likely. There's no dependable proof that eating under 1,500 mg each day of sodium is a gamble for everybody.

The body needs just a limited amount of sodium (under 500 milligrams each day) to work appropriately. That is a simple pinch — the sum in under ¼ teaspoon. Not very many individuals verge on eating, not precisely that sum. Additionally, sound kidneys are perfect for holding the sodium your body needs.

The rule to diminish to 1,500 mg may not have any significant bearing on individuals who lose enormous measures of sodium in sweat, as aggressive competitors. Laborers presented with significant intensity stress, like foundry laborers and firemen or those coordinated by their medical services supplier. There is proof that it may be destructive to specific patients with congestive cardiovascular breakdown.

On the off chance that you have ailments or other extraordinary dietary requirements or limitations, you ought to heed the guidance of a certified medical services proficient.

Chapter 5

The Salt cure

Why You Crave Salty Foods

You hunger for pungent food varieties for various reasons, frequently connected with a sodium irregularity of some sort or another. On the off chance that you will generally die for salt often, you shouldn't disregard this; salt desires could flag a more profound medical issue.

Lack of hydration

Hankering salt could mean you want to hydrate. A lack of sodium triggers hormonal frameworks that inspire desires for spicy food, and your body feels compensated when you devour savory foods.3

To prevent this from occurring, you ought to continuously keep steady throughout your daily hydration. The Establishment of Medication suggests that your total water consumption from all food varieties and fluids is 3.7 liters for men and 2.7 liters for ladies.

Do you find yourself dehydrated often? Following these tips can assist you with drinking more water:

• Convey a water bottle with you over the day, opening drinking water.

• Add a natural product or new spices to your water for flavor, empowering you to drink it regularly.

• Freeze water bottles, so you have super cold water promptly accessible.

• Request water, rather than another refreshment, while feasting out.

Addison's Disease

Addison's sickness is a problem wherein your adrenal organs don't make enough of specific chemicals, like cortisol (frequently called the pressure hormone). With this medical issue, you could require a high-sodium diet. Proficient medical services can suggest what sodium sources and how much is best for your problem.

Electrolyte Imbalance

When your electrolytes are out of balance, your body can hunger for pungent food varieties because of water lopsidedness. Electrolytes are minerals in your body that have an electric charge, as per the U.S. Public Library of Medicine.

Electrolytes are in your blood, pee, and tissues; their levels can sometimes become excessively high or excessively low. This happens when how much water you take in doesn't approach how much water you lose due to unreasonable perspiring, disorder, continuous peeing, or drinking such a large number of liquid refreshments.

Electrolytes are significant because they assist with adjusting your body's water harmony and pH levels, move supplements and waste into and out of your cells, and guarantee your nerves, muscles, and cerebrum capability to the best of your abilities.

Pregnancy

Encountering different sorts of desires during pregnancy is a peculiarity that usually happens. Such desires can incorporate pungent substances, even though inclination for and admission of savory food varieties frequently occurs in the later phases of pregnancy.

Pre-Menstruation

Ladies can encounter an expansion in food desires during pre-feminine hormonal changes, which incorporates a craving for pungent food varieties.

Boredom

Eating because of weariness is a close to home eating conduct, like pressure eating. This is a reaction to pessimistic feelings and can happen to anybody, at any weight.9 Rather than close to home eating, individuals ought to manage their pessimistic contemplations through careful eating, work out, and other significant pressure decrease methodologies, like reflection, investing energy in green spaces, and searching out significant encounters with loved ones.

Stress

You're eating conduct can rapidly be disturbed when you experience distressing circumstances. On the off chance that you will generally eat a great deal of spicy food varieties during ordinary, non-distressing times, your body could feel significantly improved when focused by eating food varieties that you ordinarily like

Foods to Prevent Salty Cravings

You can supplant sodium with sans salt substitutes without forfeiting taste. Choices incorporate the accompanying:

Citrus

Utilizing new citrus juice can light up dishes with corrosive. When a dish tastes a piece level, somewhat caustic from lemon juice can assist with making the food more satisfactory.

Herbs

Sprinkling a limited quantity of oregano on your popcorn and vegetables follows the style of Mediterranean dishes. You don't have to add excessively, as this spice can taste unpleasant with abuse.

Vinegar

As indicated by Purchaser Reports, vinegar can light up the kind of food varieties as a result of its corrosive content and act as a substitute for salt.

With zero calories and sodium, vinegar (except balsamic vinegar) can loan a generous and generally solid flavor. You can stir up the vinegar with champagne, rice wine, or white balsamic for significantly more tang.

No-Salt Seasoning Blends

You can skirt the salt and utilize a without salt flavoring mix, sold on the web and in supermarkets from different producers. A few items are accessible in a shakable container or parcel. Make certain to utilize delicately; tap just a limited quantity out of the box and save the rest for another tidbit or dinner.

You can likewise make your no-salt flavoring blend utilizing quite a few fixings, for example, onion powder, paprika, cayenne pepper, cumin, garlic powder, and dry mustard.

Garlic Salt

You can create your own lower sodium garlic salt than you purchase in stores using a three-to-one salt-to-garlic ratio, which matches in flavor to most commercial brands.

Garlic

Involving one teaspoon of new garlic for an impactful flavor instead of one teaspoon of iodized salt can dispense with up to 2,360 mg of sodium.

Carrots

Rather than crunchy popcorn bound with salt and margarine, carrots can offer a comparative surface, alongside hostile to diabetic, cholesterol-bringing down, and harmful to hypertensive wellbeing benefits.

You can buy pre-stripped little carrots, raising a significant ruckus nibble.

Potassium-Advanced Salt Substitutes

As per a concentrate in Hypertension, most people can't recognize in flavor between customary salt and potassium-improved salt substitutes containing no more prominent than 30% potassium chloride (so read the name).

The concentrate likewise notes that potassium-improved salt substitutes can hold flavor and satisfactoriness for "food acids and amino acids; umami substances; and different combinations of flavors and flavors" up to a low level of potassium chloride is used.14

The most effective method to Diminish Salt Utilization

The U.S. Food and Medication Organization (FDA) says that assuming you decrease how much sodium you devour; you can eliminate your desire for the flavoring. Making these strides can assist you with doing this:15

• Limit your utilization of bundled food varieties, particularly ones with "moment" in the name. These typically contain a robust measure of sodium.

• Set up your own lunch to bring to work, if conceivable.

• Peruse the nourishment marks to guarantee the items you consume contain in some measure under 2,300 milligrams of sodium, the suggested day to day incentive for sodium that ought not be surpassed.

• Avoid potential risk with vegetables. Stick to new, frozen with no flavoring added, or no-salt canned vegetables.

• Check protein bundles to check whether saltwater was added.

• Part entrées while eating out or promptly cut your dinner down the middle and put the food in a to-go pack to fight off eating the high measures of sodium tracked down in eatery contributions.

• Request salad dressing as an afterthought.

• Survey sodium nourishing data on an eatery's site before requesting.

End

While specific individuals could help by restricting their salt admission, a rising assortment of proof demonstrates that this approach isn't suitable for many people. To further develop general **wellbeing,** they need to begin creating suggestions in light of genuine evidence, and give people the data they and their primary care physicians need to determine what methodology turns out best for them. **Similarly,** as with the now-exposed suggestions on dietary cholesterol and fat, the sodium-hypertension fantasy appears to, fortunately, be on the exit plan. History, and purchasers, won't approve of associations that keep on gripping to their inappropriate